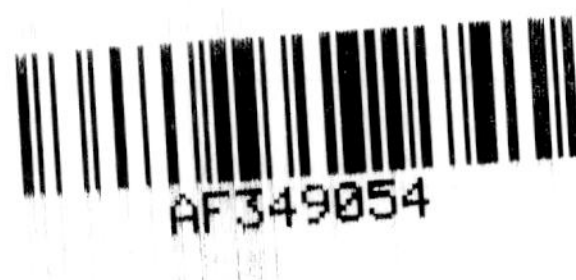
AF349054

Made in the USA
Monee, IL
07 July 2026

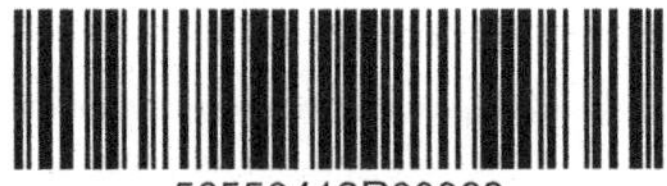

56550413R00069